AF882666

Physeo

TABLE OF CONTENTS

We would like to extend a special thanks to the following individuals who have spent many hours tutoring, guiding and consulting this work, making Physeo possible

Paloma F Cariello, MD, MPH
Assistant Professor
Division of Infectious Diseases
University of Utah School of Medicine
Salt Lake City, UT

Karen Eilbeck, Ph.D.
Professor
Biomedical Informatics
University of Utah

Vicente Planelles, Ph.D.
Professor
Division of Microbiology and Immunology
Department of Pathology
University of Utah School of Medicine
Salt Lake City, UT

Carol Foote
MD Candidate Class of 2021
University of Utah Schoold of Medicine
Salt Lake City, UT

David Ortiz
MD Candidate Class of 2021
University of Utah Schoold of Medicine
Salt Lake City, UT

Naveen Rathi
MD Candidate Class of 2021
University of Utah Schoold of Medicine
Salt Lake City, UT

PUBLIC HEALTH SCIENCES

Public Health Sciences | Section 1: Ethical Principles

I. Autonomy
   A. Autonomy is the capacity to make an informed, uncoerced decision
   B. Physician responsibility:
      1. Inform and educate the patient
      2. Honor the patient's decisions
   C. Often takes precedence in our culture

II. Beneficence
   A. Act in the patient's best interest
   B. Can sometimes conflict with autonomy or societal good

III. Nonmaleficence
   A. Do no harm
   B. Balanced with beneficence

IV. Justice
   A. Treat everyone fairly and equitably
   B. Limited by practical considerations

V. Medication Use: Introduction
   A. Unnecessary antibiotic use
   B. Opioids
   C. Nonadherence

VI. Medication Use: Unnecessary Antibiotics
   A. Insistent patient
   B. Explain that antibiotics won't help
      1. Ask for more information using open ended questions
   C. Nonmaleficence
      1. Antibiotics are not benign

VII. Medication Use: Opioid Use
   A. The opioid addict
      1. Offer alternatives and discuss treatment
      2. Can give opioids if injuries are serious
   B. The terminally ill patient
      1. Give enough opioids to ensure comfort
   C. Opioids are useful
      1. Low risk of addiction in short-term use

VIII. Medication Use: Nonadherence
   A. Attempt to identify underlying cause
   B. Provide clear instruction and work with the patient
   C. Autonomy

IX. Gifts
   A. Can be okay to accept a gift
      1. Gratitude
      2. Cultural tradition
   B. Don't accept a gift with strings attached
      1. Expectation of preferential treatment
   C. Don't accept an expensive gift
      1. Can suggest donation to charity

REVIEW QUESTIONS

1. A 63-year-old man with a history of smoking and coronary bypass surgery presents to your office for evaluation of abdominal pain. He states that he has been experiencing intense epigastric pain after eating for the past several months and that it has begun affecting his ability to eat. He thinks he has lost several pounds as a result. You suggest that the patient will need an upper endoscopy to evaluate for stomach ulcers, describing the risks and benefits of this procedure. He refuses, stating that he "hates the idea of you sticking something down my throat." He asks for a medication to help ease the pain. Which ethical principle would you be honoring by prescribing medication without performing an endoscopy? Which might you be violating?

- **The ethical principle that would be honored is autonomy. The principle that might be violating is nonmaleficence.**
- By prescribing the medication in accordance with the patient's request, the principle of autonomy is being honored.
- Prescribing medication without having a clear diagnosis, however, is a little more complicated. While this might respect the patient's autonomy, you might be violating the principle of nonmaleficence, considering you may be harming the patient by prescribing the wrong medication or not conducting a thorough evaluation.

2. A patient presents to your office for follow-up 1 month after a successful knee replacement surgery you performed for her. Her vitals are normal and her knee appears to be healing appropriately. She thanks you profusely and presents you with a beautiful handwoven scarf that she states she has been working on every day for the past month. She also knows of your love of basketball and offers you two courtside tickets to an upcoming NBA game this weekend. What should you do?

   A. Accept the gifts and thank your patient for her generosity
   B. Decline the gifts because they are too valuable and suggest that the patient could donate to charity on your behalf instead.
   C. Ask the patient why she feels it is necessary to give you such luxurious gifts.
   D. Accept the scarf but decline the basketball tickets

- **The correct answer is D.**
- Some gifts are okay for a physician to accept. In this case, the woven scarf represents a large time investment by the patient, but is not an overly expensive gift. This is an example of a gift that would be acceptable as a way to enhance the physician patient bond. However, courtside basketball tickets are usually very expensive and would likely be less appropriate for you to accept.
- A is incorrect because courtside tickets to an NBA game constitute an expensive gift that might represent a financial burden on the patient or carry a sense of obligation for the physician.
- B is incorrect because it would be appropriate to accept the scarf.
- C is incorrect because questioning a patient's motives might be considered offensive and would not be appropriate in this situation.

Public Health Sciences | Section 2: Consent and Confidentiality

I. Consent: Introduction
   A. Two major components
      1. Informed consent
      2. Consent for minors

II. Informed Consent
   A. Informed
      1. Information, understanding, capacity
   B. Consent
      1. Voluntary
   C. Exceptions
      1. Waiver
      2. Legally incompetent
      3. Emergency situations
      4. Therapeutic privilege

REVIEW QUESTIONS ?

1. 26-year-old female presents to the emergency department with increasing abdominal pain. She is diagnosed with appendicitis and informed consent is obtained for urgent surgical intervention. However, an hour later as she is being led back to the operating room, she changes her mind and decides she would rather go without surgery. As the intern on the surgical team, you explain to her the risks and benefits of the procedure again and stress the danger of delaying surgery. She expresses understanding but continues to refuse surgery. What should you do?
   A. Perform the surgery as informed consent was previously obtained
   B. Agree to delay the surgery in accordance with the patient's wishes
   C. Contact the patient's parents and spouse to obtain consent for the procedure from them
   D. Consult psychiatry to determine the patient's capacity to make this decision

- **The correct answer is B.**
- A competent patient who shows no signs of mental incapacity is within their rights to refuse treatment, even if it was considered life-saving. This patient meets the criteria for having the capacity to make decisions for herself.
- A is incorrect because she can remove her consent even after it has been previously obtained.
- B is incorrect because while her parents or spouse may be able to change her mind, she ultimately has to make the decision for herself.
- D is incorrect because there is no need to consult psychiatry to make a determination of capacity, as you are this patient's primary care team.

III. Consent for Minors
   A. Parental consent laws for minors vary by state
   B. In general, parents must consent to care
   C. Exceptions:
      1. Sex
      2. Drugs
      3. Trauma/emergencies
      4. Emancipation
   D. Encourage healthy communication and seek assent

IV. Confidentiality
   A. Vital for patient privacy and autonomy
   B. Exceptions – harm to self or others that the physician can prevent
      1. Suicidal/homicidal patient
      2. Abuse
      3. Epileptic patients – driver's license
      4. Reportable diseases (syphilis, chlamydia, etc.)

REVIEW QUESTIONS ?

2. A 2-year-old patient is brought to the emergency department by his babysitter. The patient has sustained multiple injuries to the head after falling from the top bunk of a bunk bed onto a bedside table while playing with his 4-year-old brother. His vitals are currently stable and exam shows an obviously fractured left wrist with bruising on the left side of the head. He is in a great deal of distress and won't stop crying, but appears to be okay otherwise. The babysitter has not been able to contact the parents. What should you do next?
   A. Continue to attempt to contact the parents to obtain consent before administering any treatment to the child
   B. Obtain consent for treatment from the babysitter
   C. Treat the child as if consent had been provided
   D. Perform diagnostic tests and administer pain medications but refrain from any surgical intervention until the parents can be contacted

- **The correct answer is C.**
- This situation would qualify as an emergency, and the patient could be administered reasonable treatment as if consent had been obtained.
- A is incorrect because, while attempts to contact the parents should continue, treatment should be administered regardless.
- B is incorrect because the babysitter has no legal ability to consent for the child.

REVIEW QUESTIONS

- D is incorrect because, if diagnostic tests were to reveal an intracranial bleed, surgical intervention would have to be immediately initiated. It would be inappropriate to wait for consent if the minor's life were in danger.

3. An 84-year-old woman with mild dementia presents to your office for follow-up of an infected foot ulcer. She has completed a course of antibiotics and her foot ulcer looks mostly healed. During the exam you notice that her appearance is dishevelled and she is very underweight. Upon further questioning, you learn that the patient lives with her son, but that he works very long hours and isn't home often. She cannot drive and lives in a remote area by herself. She pleads with you not to tell anyone that she is struggling as she is very embarrassed and also doesn't want her son to get in trouble for anything. What is the best course of action?

    A. Call the police and report her son for elder neglect/abuse
    B. Reassure the patient that your discussion will remain confidential
    C. Talk to the patient's son and discuss your concerns about his mother
    D. Discuss the case with your office's social worker and report the case to the appropriate state authority

- **The correct answer is D.**
- This is a case of elder neglect/abuse. The patient is clearly not being well cared for her in her current circumstance evidenced by her dishevelled appearance, infected foot ulcer, and malnourishment. This situation is a classic exception to confidentiality rules, and something must be done. It is therefore appropriate to break confidentiality and even go against the patient's will (violating her right to autonomy), in order to do what is in her best interest in accordance with the principle of beneficence.
- A is incorrect because, although it's possible that the son is intentionally neglecting his mother, it's more likely that he is busy and overwhelmed. Calling the police would be a little extreme in this circumstance. Instead, the case should be referred to the proper state authority, such as an agency that deals with protection of vulnerable populations.
- B is incorrect because the patient is in an unhealthy situation and something must be done to help her.
- C is incorrect because, although it's best to give the son the benefit of the doubt, it is not a good idea to directly confront a patient's abuser. Further help should be enlisted and the appropriate state authority must be informed.

4. A 16-year-old female presents to the emergency department with dysuria. She is diagnosed with chlamydia and gonorrhoea. She begs you to not tell her parents or her boyfriend and agrees to whatever treatment you recommend. What is the best course of action?

    A. Start treatment and agree to withhold the information from her parents, but report the infection to the health department knowing that they will contact her boyfriend
    B. Agree to keep the information confidential and start the patient on antibiotic therapy
    C. Report the infection to the health department and inform her parents and boyfriend of her diagnosis
    D. Urge the patient to tell her parents and boyfriend herself and start her on antibiotic therapy

- **The correct answer is A.**
- STIs are one of the exceptions to confidentiality when dealing with minors. While it is acceptable to withhold the information from the patient's parents, the physician must report the diagnosis to the health department knowing that they will contact her boyfriend to prevent spread of the infection.
- B is incorrect because the health department must be informed in order to stop the spread of infection and ensure the boyfriend is treated.
- C is incorrect because it is not necessary to inform the parents of the patient's diagnosis before initiating treatment.
- D is incorrect because, as mentioned above, the infection must be reported to the state health department.

Public Health Sciences | Section 3: Decision-Making Capacity

I. Capacity
   A. Introduction
      1. Capacity vs competence
         a) Capacity is a medical determination
         b) Competence is a legal determination
      2. Primary care provider determines capacity
      3. Decisions cannot be simply revoked if patient loses capacity later
   B. Determining Capacity
      1. Subjective but some general guidelines:
         a) Decisions are consistent with patient's goals and values
         b) Informed and mentally "with-it"
         c) Expresses a clear preference
         d) No clear interference by altered mental status or mood disorder
         e) Decision remains stable over time
         f) Patient is not a minor

II. Advance Directives
   A. Previously stated wish for when someone loses capacity
   B. Oral advance directive
   C. Written advance directive
      1. Living will
   D. Medical power of attorney
   E. DNR/DNI

III. Surrogate Decision Making
   A. If no advance directive exists, a surrogate decision-maker must be identified
   B. Spouse → adult children → parents → siblings → other relatives
   C. Physician can make decisions if no one else can be found
   D. Patient's best interest must be the primary consideration

REVIEW QUESTIONS

1. A 91-year-old male presents to the emergency department with severe altered mental status after being found by his neighbor on the floor. He has no clear evidence of injury, but he is somnolent and confused on the physical exam. Laboratory testing reveals that he is septic. Antibiotic therapy is initiated, but the patient continues to deteriorate and will require intubation and admission to the ICU. The neighbor isn't aware that the patient has any serious chronic health problems, but states that he thinks he remembers the patient telling him that he wouldn't want a tube down his throat and would rather die peacefully at home. You have no contact information for any of the patient's family members. What is the best course of action?

    A. Intubate the patient and transfer to the ICU for further treatment
    B. Withhold intubation and hope that antibiotics alone will be enough
    C. Stop all treatment and send the patient home
    D. Convene a hospital ethics committee to determine the best course of action

- **The correct answer is A**
- In this emergent situation and in the absence of additional information or family members, the best option is to intubate the patient and transfer him to the ICU for further treatment.
- This patient obviously does not have decision-making capacity, and the stated oral advance directive of his neighbor is not sufficient grounds upon which to withhold treatment. The neighbor is not completely sure of the patient's wishes and is not a good candidate for surrogate decision-making.
- B and C are both incorrect because the neighbor's advance directive is not reliable enough to be used as justification for withholding any life-saving treatment, whether that be intubation or antibiotic treatment.
- D is incorrect because convening a hospital ethics committee would take too long and you should be able to make the decision on your own. These types of questions will often offer the option of consulting a hospital ethics committee. This is *almost never* the correct answer, because the whole point of the question is to get you to exercise your ethical judgment.

2. 2. A 65-year-old man is hospitalized following a construction accident that involved several broken bones that were repaired surgically. He is recovering well, until post-op day 2 when he suddenly has profound chest pain and difficulty breathing. He also has altered mental status. After a few minutes, he stops breathing and you cannot find a pulse. You decide to initiate CPR before finding that he has a DNR/DNI order in his chart which was updated at the time of admission. His wife is at the bedside and states that though he may have expressed a DNR/DNI order, he didn't really mean it because he thought that he wouldn't need it until he was much older. She pleads with you to do everything you can to save her husband. What is the best course of action?

    A. Start aggressive resuscitation measures to attempt to save the patient's life
    B. Consult other family members to get a better sense of the patient's wishes
    C. Do not resuscitate the patient in accordance with the DNR/DNI
    D. Convene a hospital ethics committee to determine the best course of action

- **The correct answer is C.**
- A clear and current DNR order cannot be overruled. The patient has a clearly expressed current DNR status, and it is not for the doctor or family to determine whether it applies to this current situation or not.
- A is incorrect because the patient has a clearly expressed DNR order that was updated at the time of admission. It has to be assumed that this order is a valid expression of the patient's wishes and should not be overruled.
- B is incorrect because there is no need to go down the line of surrogate decision-makers in this case. Even the patient's spouse may not contradict the patient's clearly expressed directive, and so consulting other family members would not be appropriate.
- D is incorrect because it would take too long and you should be able to make this decision on your own. Never consult a hospital ethics committee in these types of questions.

Public Health Sciences | Section 4: Ethical Situations

I. Ethical Situations: Rapid Fire
   A. Patient concerned about radioactive food
   B. Doctor doesn't wish to prescribe emergency contraceptives for religious reasons
   C. Patient with cancer and history of opioid abuse needing pain relief
   D. Teenage male with a strong sex drive
   E. Friend who wants to be with patient despite "family only" sign
   F. Conflict between two physicians
   G. Patient wants to try alternative/holistic medicine
   H. Feeding a baby with a lethal condition
   I. Patient is victim of partner abuse
   J. Child's injuries are inconsistent with the described trauma
   K. Father objects to emergency treatment for wife and 16-year-old daughter
   L. Young child loses sister and feels guilt

REVIEW QUESTIONS

1. A 49-year-old patient presents to the emergency department complaining of a cough. You walk into the room ready to examine the patient. The patient explains to you that she is Muslim and would prefer not to be examined by a member of the opposite sex. What should you do?
   A. Explain that you are just as qualified as a female provider and that the patient should go elsewhere if that is an issue
   B. Find a female chaperone and continue with the exam
   C. Ensure the patient is stable and then refer her to a female provider who can perform the exam
   D. Skip the physical exam and treat the patient based on history and other testing

- **The correct answer is C.**
- You want to respect the autonomy of the patient by allowing her to make decisions about the care she would like to receive. However, you also want to do what is best for her and provide what care you can in accordance with the principle of beneficence. As long as she is stable, it is appropriate to refer to a female physician, rather than compromise your own standard of care or violate her stated wishes.
- A is incorrect because you should not violate the patient's autonomy by insisting that she be examined by you. If she appears stable, there is no reason for you to violate her wishes in this regard.
- B is incorrect because the patient has requested a female provider, not the presence of a chaperone.
- D is incorrect because it would be inappropriate to make a diagnosis and initiate treatment without performing a thorough physical examination.

2. A 60-year-old patient presents to the clinic demanding to have his gallbladder removed. He has been having abdominal pain for years, but has consistently had normal labs and imaging, including at this visit. You tell the patient that it is unlikely that the procedure will help with his symptoms but he insists that he have it done anyway. What is the best course of action?
   A. Refuse to perform the procedure and explain to the patient that it would be an unnecessary expense and risk to his health
   B. Refer to another physician for a second opinion
   C. Ask the patient why he thinks a cholecystectomy would be helpful
   D. Schedule a cholecystectomy after explaining the risks and benefits of the procedure

- **The correct answer is C.**
- When a patient demands a procedure that may not be necessary, it's important to approach the situation with empathy and understanding, and attempt to find out why the patient wants this particular procedure done.
- A is incorrect because an up-front refusal without attempting to understand the patient's reasoning would be inappropriate and would likely undermine your relationship with the patient.
- B is incorrect because you can make this decision on your own without requiring a referral to another physician.
- D is incorrect because you should not schedule a cholecystectomy if you truly believe the procedure to be unnecessary.

REVIEW QUESTIONS

3. A 45-year-old obese male patient presents to clinic complaining of an intense pain in his foot. On exam, you discover that the first metatarsal of his left foot is painful, swollen, and erythematous. The patient has had this condition before and has brought paperwork for you to fill out for a disabled parking permit so that he won't have to walk quite as far from his car to his office. What is the best course of action?

    A. Refuse to fill out the form and explain that with the proper treatment and lifestyle changes, the patient won't experience any more issues
    B. Fill out and submit the paperwork as the patient is clearly in need of assistance
    C. Ask the patient whether he thinks it would be ethical to get a disabled parking permit for his condition
    D. Call the Department of Motor Vehicles to ask about the policies regarding disabled parking permits

- **The correct answer is A.**
- This patient is asking for a parking permit for gout, which is an inappropriate request and should be refused.
- B is incorrect because gout is a temporary condition for which a disability claim would be unnecessary.
- C is incorrect because there is no need to ask the patient what he thinks about the situation. You should be able to explain to him that it is a temporary situation and does not qualify him as disabled or in need of a parking permit.
- D is incorrect because as the physician, you should be able to make a determination about his need for disability benefits without consulting the DMV. It's rarely the correct answer to consult with someone else when answering multiple choices questions about ethical scenarios.

4. You are rotating in a sports medicine doctor's clinic during your 3rd year clerkship rotations. As you observe the physician practice, you notice that almost every patient gets referred to an orthopedic surgeon, even for relatively minor issues. When you ask the physician about this, he explains that he has an agreement with the surgeon that benefits the practice financially for every patient he refers. He tells you not to worry because the surgeon only performs surgeries that are absolutely necessary. What is the best course of action?

    A. Report this physician to the state licensure board as he is accepting unethical kickbacks for referring patients inappropriately
    B. Express concern and encourage the physician to at least disclose this arrangement with his patients so that they are aware of this potential conflict of interest
    C. Do nothing, as medicine is a business and arrangements like this are common
    D. Call the surgeon's office and urge them to end this arrangement

- **The correct answer is B.**
- This physician's actions, while not overtly harming patients, are not ethical. In this case, encouraging the physician to at least disclose this arrangement with his patients would be the best course of action.
- A is incorrect because reporting the physician to the licensure board would be an extreme reaction to this behavior, although it would be appropriate in situations where the physician's actions were dangerous.
- C is incorrect because in this situation, it is incumbent upon you to do something despite the imbalance of power between you and the physician. Business arrangements like this may be common, but if you observe a high volume of referrals even for minor complaints, then you should act to protect the interests of the patients.
- D is incorrect because the situation should be addressed with the physician with whom you are acquainted. You should avoid going behind the physician's back to address the issue with his colleague.

REVIEW QUESTIONS

5. A 26-year-old patient presents to the emergency department after sustaining significant trauma in a motor vehicle accident. He is in hypovolemic shock and requires a blood transfusion. However, he declines this intervention as he is a Jehovah's Witness and it contradicts his religious beliefs. What should you do?

   A. Transfuse the patient as his condition is life-threatening and the situation is an emergency
   B. Find out more about the patient's beliefs and attempt to explain to him the importance of the blood transfusion, but do not transfuse against the patient's wishes
   C. Call the patient's family to have them convince him to accept this intervention
   D. Consult the hospital ethics board to determine whether or not the patient should be transfused

- **The correct answer is B.**
- In this case, the patient shows no signs of lacking capacity and has refused a life-saving intervention. Although he is likely to die without it, he is able to refuse this intervention and his decision should be respected.
- A is incorrect because the patient is a competent adult and can decide to refuse a life-saving intervention.
- C is incorrect because calling the patient's family to have them convince him to change his mind would not be respectful of the patient's autonomy and would violate patient-doctor confidentiality.
- D is incorrect because, as usual, it is not necessary to involve the hospital ethics board in a straightforward case of a competent patient refusing care.

6. A 75-year-old patient has test results that indicate she has a terminal condition with a life expectancy of less than 6 months. Her family asks you not to disclose any test results that indicate a poor prognosis, as they don't think the patient will be able to handle it. What is the best course of action?

   A. Withhold the test results from the patient in accordance with the family's wishes
   B. Explain that you must divulge the test results to the patient as long as she has decision making capacity
   C. Attempt to understand why the patient's family would like to withhold this information from the patient and then make a decision based on this information
   D. Repeat testing to ensure that your results are valid

- **The correct answer is C.**
- It's important to remember that you must disclose any relevant health information to the patient in almost every circumstance. The only situations in which it might be appropriate to withhold information is (a) if the patient is not competent/lacks capacity, or (b) if you need to invoke therapeutic privilege because you believe the information may cause the patient to harm himself/herself/themselves or others. In this case, it is not appropriate to blindly accept the family's wishes. However, it is appropriate to get more information from the patient's family to determine whether the patient either lacks capacity or is at risk of harming herself or others.
- A is incorrect because more information should be obtained before deciding whether or not to acquiesce to the family's wishes in this situation.
- B is incorrect because in the case of therapeutic privilege, it may be appropriate to withhold information from the patient.
- D is incorrect because there is no reason to suspect that your test results are invalid, and therefore there is no reason to repeat them.

REVIEW QUESTIONS

7. A 15-year-old patient presents to your clinic with a positive pregnancy test, hoping to establish prenatal care. Her parents have accompanied the patient and brought adoption paperwork, insisting that the patient begin preparing to put the child up for adoption. Your patient is adamant that she would like to keep the child and raise her. What is the best course of action?

   A. Respect the patient's wishes and refrain from participating in any preparation for adoption
   B. Attempt to help persuade the patient that adoption is the best course of action as she is underage and a child would likely represent a significant burden
   C. Present all options to the patient including termination of the pregnancy
   D. Fill out the adoption paperwork as the patient is underage and therefore her parents have legal decision-making authority over her

- The correct answer is A
- Mothers have the right to make decisions regarding their babies unless they're judged to lack capacity or ability to care for them. While parents of minors generally make medical decisions on their behalf, the minor in this question still has decision making capacity for her child. While it is appropriate to provide more information to the patient, you should respect the patient's wishes and refrain from participating in any preparation for adoption.
- B is incorrect because It is also inappropriate to attempt to persuade the patient to pursue any specific course of action, especially in the case where the patient might feel ganged up on by you and her parents.
- C is incorrect because it is likely that the patient is aware of her options and in this situation, you must serve as her advocate and not jeopardize your relationship with her by presenting her with options which could be interpreted as an attempt to change her mind.
- D is incorrect because, as previously mentioned, persons under age 18 have the decision making capacity for their own children and the parents are not legally authorized to decide the fate of the baby. In this case, it is important to above all respect the patient's autonomy and right to make this decision for herself.

8. An attractive 26-year-old female patient repeatedly presents to your office complaining of breast tenderness. You have performed multiple physical examinations with imaging and laboratory testing with no significant results. The patient thanks you and states that she feels reassured to have such an incredible doctor taking care of her. She asks if she can take you to dinner to express her gratitude. What is the best course of action?

   A. Accept the invitation as an appropriate expression of the patient's gratitude
   B. Attempt to clarify with the patient whether she is asking you on a date or whether the dinner will respect your physician-patient relationship
   C. Politely decline the invitation as it is unethical to enter into a romantic relationship with this patient
   D. Accept the invitation but first transfer care of the patient to a different physician as it is acceptable to date former but not current patients

- **The correct answer is C.**
- While dating a patient is generally not illegal, it's still unethical. There is some nuance involved in these scenarios, as it is technically okay to date a former patient. The AMA guidelines state that "sexual or romantic relationships with former patients are unethical if the physician uses or exploits trust, knowledge, emotions, or influence derived from the previous professional relationship, or if a romantic relationship would otherwise foreseeably harm the individual."
- A is incorrect because there is clearly more going on here than a simple expression of the patient's gratitude, and dinner would likely lead to the development of a potentially inappropriate relationship.
- B is incorrect because there is no need to ask the patient what her intentions are. There is nothing to be gained from asking this patient what her intentions are, and a decision should be made based on the information offered in the vignette.
- D is incorrect because, while you could transfer care to another physician and still technically date the patient, there are a few indications from the question stem (such as repeat breast exam requests and praising the physician) that suggest that perhaps there may be a potential power imbalance or emotional influence derived from the physician-patient relationship that would make any romantic relationship inappropriate.

REVIEW QUESTIONS

9. You are an oncologist working in a hectic outpatient clinic and you accidently perform a bone marrow biopsy on the wrong patient. What should you do?

    A. Provide free medical care to that patient for the next year to compensate for the mistake
    B. Explain to the patient that an error occurred but do not admit fault because to do so would risk unnecessary liability
    C. Explain to the patient exactly what happened as you understand it and apologize for your error
    D. Monitor for any adverse effects, but do not disclose the error because the patient will likely experience minimal harm from this mistake

- **The correct answer is C.**
- In the case of medical error, you have to be upfront and disclose the error. Never attempt to cover it up or dodge responsibility for your mistakes, even if no direct harm was caused to the patient.
- A is incorrect because there is no need to provide free medical care to the patient as compensation for the mistake. This would not necessarily be an inappropriate form of compensation, but the most important first step here is to explain what happened and apologize.
- B is incorrect because as previously stated, you must be upfront and admit responsibility for your mistakes, despite liability concerns.
- D is incorrect because the outcome of mistakes should not dictate your behavior in relation to disclosing and apologizing for them.

10. You notice another physician in your practice appears intoxicated. The previous week a patient that usually sees this physician presented to you for another issue, and you noticed that the patient had been prescribed the wrong dose of a medication. What is the best course of action?

    E. Confront your colleague and see what you can do to help
    F. Report your colleague's behavior to a supervisor and have them investigate the issue formally
    G. Do nothing as your partner is an adult and is responsible for their own actions
    H. Report your colleague's behavior to the state licensing board and recommend license suspension

- **The correct answer is B.**
- While conflict between physicians is generally best handled with a direct two-way conversation, in a case where the physician is impaired and this impairment has caused harm to patients, you are obligated to report the situation to the appropriate supervisory personnel.
- A is incorrect because while it may be appropriate to offer counsel to your colleague, your duty is primarily to protect and serve patients, and therefore a physician who represents a threat to patients should be reported.
- C is incorrect because it is incumbent upon you to put the interest of patients first and report your colleague's potentially harmful actions.
- D is incorrect because a resolution should first be sought from your supervisors. If the situation is not resolved by local supervisors, then it would be appropriate to report your colleague to the state licensing board.

Public Health Sciences | Section 5: Geriatrics

I. Physiological Changes
   A. Dulled senses
      1. Presbyopia: lens stiffens
      2. Presbycusis: loss of hair cells
   B. Diminished immune response
   C. Decreased renal, pulmonary, GI function
      1. GFR = 100 – 10 per decade after age 40
   D. Muscle → fat
      1. Weight-bearing exercise
   E. Sleep changes:
      1. Decreased sleep latency
      2. Decreased REM
      3. Wake up early

II. Sexual Changes
   A. Men
      1. Slow erection, delayed ejaculation
      2. Longer refractory period, decreased libido
   B. Women
      1. Vaginal shortening, wall thinning, dryness
      2. Decreased libido

III. Psychological/Social Changes
   A. Depression/suicide
      1. Social isolation, poor health
   B. Intelligence remains largely the same
      1. Fluid intelligence
      2. Crystallized intelligence

IV. Elder Abuse
   A. Vulnerable population
      1. Health issues, social isolation
   B. Mistreatment by caregiver
   C. Neglect
   D. Abandonment
   E. Exploitation
   F. Legal responsibility

REVIEW QUESTIONS

1. An 85 year-old-man is brought to the clinic by his daughter who is concerned that he is "not as sharp as he used to be." She states that he has had difficulty remembering his grandchildren's names, he struggles to find the right words in conversations, and he often only responds to his name after it is repeatedly called. She also reports that he has had more difficulty getting around lately and is having to use his cane more frequently than before. Examination reveals a pleasant, elderly man who is not concerned about his cognitive ability. He scores 26/30 on a mini-mental status exam and has no neurologic deficits. What is the best course of action?

    A. Prescribe an SSRI for depression-related cognitive decline
    B. Obtain brain imaging to screen for normal-pressure hydrocephalus
    C. Reassure the patient's daughter that he is experiencing normal cognitive decline related to aging
    D. Diagnose the patient with Alzheimer disease and prescribe donepezil

- **The correct answer is C.**
- The patient is experiencing normal cognitive decline related to aging supported by the results of his mini-mental status exam. A score of 24 or greater is considered normal, and this patient scored 26 out of 30. His gait difficulties are also easily explained by his advanced age.
- A is incorrect although an SSRI would be a reasonable solution for a depressed patient. Although depression can cause significant cognitive decline this patient does not meet the SIGECAPS depression criteria based on his history.
- B is incorrect because the patient doesn't have symptoms consistent with normal-pressure hydrocephalus. Normal-pressure hydrocephalus is characterized by cognitive decline combined with incontinence and gait difficulty (a "wide-based" gait). Getting an MRI would be appropriate if you suspected this condition, but this patient's cognitive decline is not quite severe enough to cause concern.
- D is incorrect because, given the mild nature of his cognitive decline, Alzheimer's would not be an appropriate diagnosis.

2. An 86-year-old female with multiple serious health conditions presents to the clinic with a broken arm and several bruises around her wrists and on her face. She is tearful and mumbles something about falling down the stairs. After further questioning, she admits that the injuries were caused by her husband who has a short temper and sometimes directs this anger towards her. She states that her many health problems have become a significant burden for him and this likely accounts for his increased stress. She begs you not to tell anyone about what she told you, as she would be "destitute" if her husband left her. What is the best course of action?

    A. Immediately call Adult Protective Services and report the husband for elder abuse
    B. Treat the patient's injuries and reassure her that your discussion will remain confidential
    C. Talk to the patient's husband and seek support for him to help relieve the burden of caring for his wife
    D. Call the police to arrest the patient's husband for his assault

- **The correct answer is A.**
- While there is no federal law requiring the reporting of elder abuse, all states have laws that require physicians to immediately report suspected elder abuse. In this scenario, it's helpful to recognize that in order to ensure this patient's safety, her autonomy must be violated and you must not comply with her request to keep the information confidential.
- B is incorrect for the reasons stated immediately above.
- C is incorrect because it is important to remove the victim from her abusive circumstance. While it's possible that her husband might need support, providing family counseling in this case is not the role of the physician.
- D is incorrect because calling the police would be too extreme in this case, and adult protective services should be consulted first.

Public Health Sciences | Section 6: Developmental Milestones

I. Gross Motor
   A. Lifts head – 1 month
   B. Rolls over – 4 months
   C. Sits up unsupported – 6 months
   D. Crawls – 8 months
   E. Stands – 10 months
   F. Walks – 12-18 months
   G. Runs – 2 years
   H. Tricycle – 3 years
   I. Hops on one foot – 4 years

II. Fine Motor
   A. Eyes track objects – 2 months
   B. Pass object from hand to hand – 6 months
   C. Pincer grasp – 10 months
   D. Points at objects – 1 year
   E. Stacking blocks – (3 x age in years)
   F. Feeds self with cutlery – 20 months
   G. Copies line/circle/cross/square – 2/3/4/5 years
   H. Triangles and diamonds - >5 years
   I. Buttons/zippers – 5 years

III. Social
   A. Social smile – 2 months
   B. Orients to voice/name – 4 months/9 months
   C. Stranger anxiety – 6 months
   D. Separation anxiety – 9 months
   E. Rapprochement – 1-2 years
   F. Parallel play – 2-3 years
   G. Gender identity/sex curiosity – 3 years
   H. Comfortable spending part of day away from mother – 3 years
   I. Friends, real/imaginary – 4 years

IV. Language
   A. Babbling – 4-6 months
   B. Repetitive responding (mama, dada) – 10 months
   C. 10 words – 1 year
   D. 200 words, 2-word sentences, parents understand child – 2 years
   E. 1000 words, strangers understand child (around ¾) – 3 years
   F. Can tell stories – 4 years

V. Cognition
   A. Sensorimotor stage – 0-2 years
   B. Object permanence (peek-a-boo) – 7 months
   C. Pre-operational phase – 2-7 years
   D. Pretend play, symbols
   E. Concrete operational phase – 7-11 years
   F. Conservation
   G. Formal operational phase – 12+ years

REVIEW QUESTIONS

1. A 2-year-old girl is brought to the clinic by her father for evaluation. She was born with multiple birth defects and has significant cognitive delay. So far, she has not started walking and instead mostly crawls to get around. She has recently started pulling herself up to a standing position using chairs. She cannot use cutlery but has also recently started eating cheerios out of a bag on her own. She has achieved milestones normally reached by a child of what age?

- **A 10-month-old child with normal development.**
- In this question, we are presented with a developmentally delayed child who recently started pulling herself to a standing position and using a pincer grasp to eat cheerios. These milestones are characteristic of a 10-month-old child with normal development.
- However, this child is 2-years-old; which would mean that she is about 14 months delayed overall.

REVIEW QUESTIONS

2. A mother brings her 17-month-old son to the clinic for a routine check-up. In the office, you observe him mostly crawling around, occasionally pulling himself upright while hanging onto chairs on the examination table. You observe him happily playing with and stacking some blocks. He points to things around the room to show his mom, exclaiming "mama look!" but won't talk to you and runs to his mother when you try to engage with him. What is the most likely diagnosis?

    A. Fine motor developmental delay
    B. Gross motor developmental delay
    C. Normal development
    D. Language developmental delay

- **The correct answer is C.**
- This question is pretty straightforward but also fairly typical of what you might see on Step 1.
- It should be pretty easy to see that this child is on-track and is meeting all of his developmental milestones. He's able to stack some blocks, says a few words, and demonstrates appropriate shyness towards you; the physician.
- The only domain in which he may be experiencing some difficulty is in gross motor, as he is not yet walking. However, the cut-off for diagnosing a delay in being able to walk is 18 months so this child still has another month and he appears to be getting there, as evidenced by his pulling himself up to a stand.

3. 3. A father brings in his 30-month-old daughter to the office. He is concerned that she may have autism. He states that she is very quiet and is hard to understand when she does speak. He has also noticed that she doesn't interact much with other children. Even when play-dates have been arranged with friends, she mostly plays with toys by herself. You observe her in the office happily playing with blocks. She picks one up to show you and smiles. What is the best course of action?

    E. Refer to a specialist for autism screening
    F. Conduct a hearing screening test
    G. Enroll the child in speech therapy
    H. Reassurance

- **The correct answer is B.**
- The child presented in this case appears to have a language delay as she isn't speaking much and is difficult to understand. She does not appear delayed in other domains as she plays with blocks and the father's description of her playing behavior seems to describe parallel play, which is appropriate for her age.
- In a patient such as this, it's important to screen them for hearing difficulties before initiating any intervention. Because hearing and speech appear to be the only thing this child has difficulty with, a hearing screening test would be a reasonable place to start.
- A is incorrect because autism is unlikely given the child's interaction with the physician in the office, where she responds appropriately to social interaction.
- C is incorrect because although she may indeed need speech therapy, it's important to conduct a hearing screening test first to determine whether she has any hearing deficits that could be causing her speech issues.
- D would also be inappropriate given this patient does have a significant language delay

Public Health Sciences | Section 7: Healthcare Delivery

I. Disease Prevention
   A. Primary
      1. Prevent disease from occurring (vaccination, hand-washing)
   B. Secondary
      1. Screening to catch disease early (pap smear)
   C. Tertiary
      1. Treatment (chemotherapy)
   D. Quaternary
      1. Protecting patients from harm of unnecessary intervention

Health Plan	PCP Required	Network	Other Features
Health Maintenance Organization (HMO)	- Yes	- Must be in-network	- Must have a referral to see specialist - Cheaper
Point of Service (POS)	- Yes	- Can see out-of-network (at higher cost)	- Must have a referral to see specialist - More expensive
Preferred Provider Organization (PPO)	- No	- Open Network	- Higher copays and deductibles - More expensive
Exclusive Provider Organization (EPO)	- No	- Very limited network - Much more expensive if out-of-network care is sought	- Cheaper

TABLE 10.1.1 - Types of Health Plans

II. Payment Models
   A. Fee for service
      1. Criticized for providing perverse incentives
   B. Bundled payment
      1. Certain amount of money for a set period of time
   C. Capitation
      1. Similar to bundled payment except tied to each individual patient
   D. Global payment
      1. Set payment for procedures

III. Medicare
   A. > 65-years-old, dialysis, disabled for > 2 years
   B. Four parts
      1. A: Hospital and hospice care
      2. B: Basic medical bills
      3. C: A+B by private insurance partner
      4. D: Prescription drugs

IV. Medicaid
   A. Patients under a certain income level (poverty line)
   B. Pregnant patients
   C. Children

V. Hospice
   A. End of life care that prioritizes comfort and palliation
   B. <6 months life expectancy
   C. Opioids, sedatives, anxiolytics
   D. Not assisted suicide

VI. Common Causes of Death
   A. Infants <1: birth defects, preterm, SIDS
   B. Ages 1-14: **accidents**, cancer, birth defects
   C. Ages 15-34: **accidents**, suicide, homicide
   D. Ages 35-44: **accidents**, cancer, heart disease
   E. Ages 45-64: cancer, heart disease, unintentional injury
   F. Ages 65+: heart disease, cancer, COPD

VII. Re-hospitalization
   A. Medicare: CHF, septicemia, pneumonia
   B. Medicaid: mood disorders, schizophrenia/psychosis, diabetes
   C. Uninsured: mood disorders, alcohol-related disorders, diabetes
   D. Private insurance: chemotherapy, mood disorders, complications from surgical procedures

REVIEW QUESTIONS

1. You are working on a research project with the radiology department to develop a new screening test for lung cancer that would detect it with greater accuracy earlier in its course. The test does occasionally yield false positive results, leading to unnecessary biopsy and treatment. However, your research principal investigator hopes that implementing this test will give physicians a tool that they can use to more effectively counsel their patients to quit smoking. What type of prevention would this screening test constitute?

   A. Primary prevention
   B. Secondary prevention
   C. Tertiary prevention
   D. Quaternary prevention

- **The correct answer is A.**
- This question has a couple of distractors to complicate the picture but at its core, the screening test is an attempt to detect a disease early on and prevent it from getting worse.
- One of the distractors in this stem is in the form of the research PI hoping that the test will allow physicians to counsel patients to quit smoking more effectively.
- Having patients quit smoking is a form of primary prevention as it prevents the negative effects of smoking.
- Another potential distractor is that the test leads to some unnecessary treatment so it could be argued that eliminating the test would be a form of quaternary prevention: helping to keep patients from experiencing harm caused by the medical system.

2. A 76-year-old patient on medicare is admitted to the hospital for treatment of a malignant lung adenocarcinoma. He is initiated on chemotherapy and remains in the hospital for 2 weeks. He does not work with a private insurer. Under what part of medicare will his chemotherapy drugs be covered?

   A. Part A
   B. Part B
   C. Part C
   D. Part D

- **The correct answer is A**
- Although the patient is being treated with chemotherapy drugs, which you were told are covered under medicare part D, ALL hospital inpatient care is covered under medicare part A. Anything that has to do with hospital or hospice, including drugs used inpatient, is covered by part A.
- B is incorrect because part B of medicare covers medical bills such as doctor's office visits and procedures, not hospital expenses.
- C is incorrect because part C of medicare is a combination of parts A and B handled by private insurance, which the question specifically states is not the case of this patient.
- D is incorrect because although chemotherapy drugs are drugs, hospital expenses are all covered by part A of medicare.

REVIEW QUESTIONS

3. A 92-year-old patient is started on home hospice. Prior to this, an end-of-life care discussion with her family is conducted wherein she expresses a desire to be lucid and able to communicate with the family as long as possible. About 2 months into hospice care, she has waxing and waning levels of consciousness and is complaining of significant pain. She is already on a moderately high dose of an opioid medication. Her adult son is at the bedside and requests pain medication to help ease his mother's pain. What is the best course of action?

   A. Administer a higher dose of morphine
   B. Withhold pain medication to help sharpen the patient's mental status
   C. Initiate delirium protocol and eliminate unnecessary medications
   D. Administer naloxone as the patient has likely overdosed on opioids

- **The correct answer is A.**
- The key to answering this question is remembering that the purpose of hospice is to ensure the comfort of the patient. Although the patient expressed a desire to remain lucid as long as possible, treating the pain is the highest priority. Mental status would be expected to deteriorate at the end of life and the fact that this patient is in hospice means that this is an expected development.
- B is incorrect because although the patient expressed a desire to remain as lucid as possible, the primary goal of hospice is to provide maximum comfort for this patient. Therefore, it would be inappropriate to withhold pain medication in this instance.
- C is incorrect because even if the patient is suffering from delirium, she is nearing the end of her life and you should prioritize her pain treatment above all else.
- D is incorrect because the patient has not clearly overdosed on opioids and is continuing to complain of significant pain, which should be treated.

Public Health Sciences | Section 8: Quality and Safety

I. Safety Culture
   A. An environment where everyone is responsible for patient safety
      1. No fear of censure for reporting events
      2. Can be difficult in a hierarchical system
   B. Must have event reporting systems for review

II. Human Factors Design
   A. System designed to minimize potential for human error
   B. Forcing functions
      1. Patient with a documented allergy in EMR - are you sure?
   C. Standardization
      1. Checklists, guidelines, algorithms
   D. Simplification
      1. Automatic calculator

III. PDSA Cycle
   A. Plan – identify problem and propose solution
   B. Do – test it out
   C. Study – analyze results
   D. Act – implement solution into new workflow

IV. Quality Measurements
   A. Structural - equipment, resources, facilities
   B. Process - system performance as planned
   C. Outcome - impact on patients
   D. Balancing - impact on other systems/outcomes

V. Swiss Cheese Model
   A. Multiple safeguards
   B. Errors are a systems issue
   C. "Near miss" events

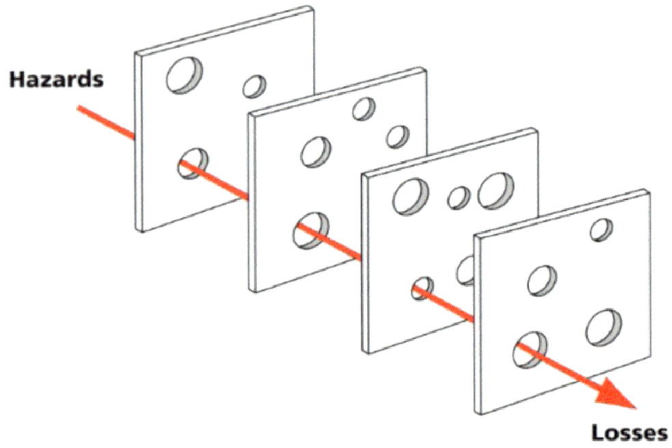

FIGURE 10.1.1 - Swiss Cheese Model

VI. Swiss Cheese Model: Example
   A. Administering the wrong drug to a patient
   B. Multiple safeguards
      1. Pharmacist enters prescription information into the EMR
      2. Pharmacist double checks the label
      3. Nurse checks the label against EMR
      4. Nurse scans the barcode
   C. If even one step is carried out, the medical error is prevented

VII. Types of Medical Errors
   A. Active error
      1. Actively committed
      2. Errors of neglect or omission
   B. Latent error
      1. Accidents waiting to happen
   C. Should be disclosed regardless of outcome

VIII. Medical Error Analysis
   A. Root-cause analysis
      1. Retrospective approach
      2. After an error
   B. Failure mode and effects analysis
      1. Forward-looking (prospective) approach
      2. Predicting failure

REVIEW QUESTIONS

1. You are a surgical resident providing post-operative care to an elderly man who has just undergone a hip replacement operation. You prescribe him a high dose of oxycodone to help with his significant postoperative pain. While you are signing this prescription, the computer asks you to verify your credential. You do so and the computer then requires you to review the patient's information and enter their patient MRN to ensure you are prescribing opioids to the right patient. Which of the following best describes the information above?

    A. Standardization of care
    B. Forced function
    C. Simplification
    D. Dual authentication

- **The correct answer is B.**
- The process described in this vignette should come across as a pretty clear example of forced function. Before prescribing this potentially dangerous medication, you are being required by the computer system to verify that you are prescribing it to the correct patient. This is a classic example of forced function, requiring someone to make sure they are doing something correctly and not allowing them to do it on autopilot.
- A is incorrect because standardization of care refers to implementing protocols to allow for the best evidence-based practices to be incorporated into each patient's care.
- C is incorrect because an EMR asking for patient verification is not an example of simplification.
- D is incorrect because dual authentication is not a widely recognized design label to help control for human error.

2. You are a medical student rotating on an internal medicine service. You are given responsibility for a patient admitted for exacerbation of COPD. While going through your patient's chart, you notice that he has not been receiving his outpatient antipsychotic medication for the past week of his hospitalization. When you mention this to your resident he says, "Whoops! Good catch. I will add that back now." What should you do next?

    A. Let it go as there was no clear harm done
    B. Recommend reporting the lapse to the administration
    C. Remind your resident to be more diligent in the future
    D. Conduct a root-cause analysis to determine how this occurred
    E. Inform the patient and apologize for the lapse and recommend reporting the error to the administration

- **The correct answer is E.**
- This is a medical error that caused no clear harm to the patient but would be classified as a "near miss event" and is still valuable to analyze from a systems perspective. However, as a medical student, it is not necessarily appropriate to report your resident without discussing the matter with him first. The key to answering this question is recognizing that with any medical error, it is essential that you inform the patient, regardless of the outcome.
- A is incorrect because an event like this should be reported for quality improvement purposes even if no harm was caused in this particular instance.
- B is incorrect because it doesn't mention informing the patient, a key step in addressing the mistake.
- C is incorrect because while you may want to remind your resident to be more diligent in the future, you must report the event and inform the patient in addition.
- D is incorrect because it is not your responsibility as a medical student to conduct a root-cause analysis. You are responsible for reporting an error and allowing the administration the opportunity to conduct a root-cause analysis of the mistake.

TABLES & FIGURES

Made in the USA
Las Vegas, NV
03 November 2026

57424359R00017